Negotiating Terms of Employment

Carolyn Buppert

A publication of the
LAW OFFICE OF CAROLYN BUPPERT

Annapolis, Maryland
2006

This publication is designed to provide accurate and authoritative information regarding the subject matter covered. It is sold with the understanding that the publisher, who renders legal services to individual clients, is, in this book, commenting only on the situations described herein, and is not providing advice to individual readers about situations which may be factually or legally dissimilar to the cases addressed in the book. If legal advice or other expert assistance is required by a reader, the services of a qualified attorney should be sought. Sound legal advice depends upon an analysis of the facts specific to a situation, analysis of relevant state and federal law, and an application of the facts of a situation to the law.

ISBN 0-9722476-2-9
Library of Congress Control Number: 2002095334

For information on copying or use of this material:
Carolyn Buppert
Law Office of Carolyn Buppert
1419 Forest Dr., Suite 205
Annapolis, MD 21403.

Orders: Use the form on the last page of this book
and mail to the address above.

Table of contents

PREFACE

The principles of negotiation are the same, whether the participants are nurse practitioner and medical practice owner, professional basketball player and team owner, or lawmaker and citizen advocate.

These are:

- Ask for what you want. If you don't ask for it, you aren't likely to get it.
- Have something to offer. If you don't deserve what you want, you aren't likely to get it.
- Justify your request. Even if you ask for something, and deserve it, you aren't likely to get it unless you are successful at convincing the other party that they should part with their money, their time or their vote.

To be successful at negotiating, an individual must:

- Know what he or she wants, and be able to articulate it.
- Describe what he or she has to offer.
- Know what the other party wants or, at minimum, have a sense of what the other party wants.
- Be able to articulate why what the individual has to offer

fits with what the other party wants. Or, if the fit is questionable, articulate how the parties might accommodate each other's needs in some mutually beneficial way.

An attorney who represents professional athletes in negotiations with team owners says successful negotiations depend on 3 P's: Prepare, Probe and Propose.

This book addresses the principles of negotiation and applies them to negotiating employment as a nurse practitioner. Part 1 addresses the who, what, where, when and why of negotiation. Part 2 addresses the "hows" of negotiating: preparing, give and take, and closing the negotiations. Part 3 addresses the contract language.

PART 1

Negotiating: Who, what, where, when and why

Situation A: Pediatrician wants the 5 NPs working at his practice to be bound by an employment contract.

Dr. Black employs 5 NPs — Flowers, who has been with him 17 years, Grass and Tree, who have been with him part-time for 10 years and Rock and Stone, who have been with him a year or less. On June 15, Dr. Black presents all 5 NPs with a 23-page document drafted by his attorney. Dr. Black says "I want this signed by July 1. Starting July 1, I will be paying all of you a percentage of collections attributable to you, rather than a set salary. All of you get the same contract, but there are provisions for higher percentages for those of you who have been with me the longest. We'll meet about this next Thursday at 7 p.m."

The NPs read the contract, which states that they will be paid somewhere between 31% and 37% of collections for their services. The new NPs — Rock and Stone — will be paid 31% of collections and the most senior NP — Flowers — will be paid 37% of collections. Grass and Tree, the NPs who have 10 years of experience, will be paid 33% of collections. All benefits and practice expenses attributable to the NPs (such as health insurance and continuing education expenses) will be deducted from the total collections, and the NPs' paychecks will reflect the difference between collections and expenses. They still will get paychecks every two weeks, but it is "an advance on a draw" rather than a clean payment. At the end of each quarter, the revenues generated and expenses incurred by each NP will be compared, and each will either get an additional check or be required to return money already advanced.

The contract includes the following clause: "Nurse practitioner will not, upon leaving Black Group, for any reason, accept employment or practice in pediatrics within a 10 mile radius of any Black Group practice location for a period of one year following termination. Should the nurse practitioner violate this covenant not to compete, the nurse practitioner agrees to pay all of Black Group's attorneys' fees spent in order to enforce this clause."

The NPs confer and decide to meet with an attorney.

Situation #B: Endocrinologist White wants to hire an NP.

Dr. White has always been a sole practitioner. NP Waters has just completed a master's degree program qualifying him as a nurse practitioner. NP Waters needs a job. Neither Endocrinologist White nor NP Waters have the faintest idea how to construct an employment agreement, or even if one is desirable or necessary.

The basics:

Just about everything is negotiable, given the right circumstances. A binding agreement consists of a promise made in return for something of value. For example, an employee promises to work and, in return, an employer promises to pay salary. Before people make promises, there is often much discussion — negotiation — about who will give what in return for what.

NPs may be negotiating with

- employers or potential employers
- co-workers
- hospital or nursing home administrators
- conference organizers
- publishers
- insurance companies or managed care organizations
- pharmaceutical companies
- medical societies
- lawmakers
- bureaucrats, or
- patients.

The issues which a nurse practitioner might negotiate include:

- salary
- benefits
- working conditions, including hours, number of assistants, on-call services
- bonus
- terms for handling matters after an NP leaves a practice
- terms under which an NP speaks at a conference or writes an article for publication
- terms under which an NP consults with a university, program, agency or facility

- the fee schedule for specific CPT codes
- a capitated fee schedule
- language of a bill before a legislative body
- language of a regulation promulgated by the Medicare agency
- terms for a vendor's exhibit at an educational conference
- terms for publishing of a manuscript
- terms under which an NP will see a patient, or
- who will cover call this weekend.

Negotiations may take place at a scheduled date, time and place or may be conducted informally, piece by piece, over a long term. The parties each may have an attorney, or not. NPs may negotiate together with other NPs in the group, or individually. They may negotiate with all of the partners in a practice, or a designated negotiator. The negotiations may lead to a written contract, or may be agreed upon orally.

Why negotiate? Because it is rare that two people's wants and needs are perfectly apparent and perfectly synchronized. Often, through a process of give and take, people make compromises which provide most of their needs and wants.

Part 2

Negotiating: How

Preparing

A nurse practitioner, or anyone else, prepares to negotiate by a) determining what he or she wants, b) prioritizing wants and needs, c) determining what he or she can offer, d) determining what the other party wants, and e) analyzing the fit between what the NP wants and what the other party wants.

If an NP is employed "at will" (see Part 3 for a discussion of "at will" employment) and wants to negotiate a contract with the current employer, the preparation is done over the course of the year preceding the negotiations. If an NP is seeking a new job, the preparation is done in two parts. The first part of data collection is done at the NP's current job. The NP wants to provide the prospective employer with data on the NP's ability to generate revenues. So, an NP collects data on his or her productivity — patient procedures or visits conducted, revenues generated, non-monetary assets brought to the practice — at the current job. (If the NP is a recent graduate, and has no data on productivity, the NP may project productivity data, as long as the NP makes it clear that the numbers are projections, not facts.) The second part of data collection aims at gathering information on the prospective employer. This is done during the application and interview process.

Determining what you want

If you've worked your way through an educational program for nurse practitioners, it is likely that you have faced, are facing or will be facing negotiations for employment. If you are currently practicing, chances are good that you and your employer will want to negotiate some aspect of your relationship, if not now, then in the future.

Either way, think about this question: "What makes for a 'good day' at work?" It makes little sense to devote 8 or more hours a day to solving other people's problems if that isn't satisfying in some way. A nurse practitioner might decide that it makes his or her day to

- design and implement a system to track patient follow-up, thereby avoiding malpractice
- efficiently process large numbers of patients, knowing he or she will be rewarded for a high rate of billings
- be greeted on the street by patients who announce proudly to their friends "This is my child's nurse practitioner!"
- be introduced at a conference as a well-regarded expert on some clinical issue, or
- prove or disprove a clinical hypothesis.

An individual who knows what drives himself or herself will be able, over time, to build the knowledge, experience and connections to maximize satisfying experiences.

First, ask yourself "What do I really like to do?" Then, look at the job. An audit tool for rating one's current job is provided as Appendix A. A brief, general self-assessment tool, addressing "wants" unrelated to the current job is provided in Appendix B.

Considering the answers you gave to the questions in the Appendices, what are your

Must haves?

1. ______________________________
Example: Salary of $70,000+ a year

2. ______________________________
Example: Health insurance

3. ______________________________
Example: Opportunity to develop specific expertise

Would likes?

1. ______________________________
Example: Opportunity for bonus

2. ______________________________
Example: Training to perform colposcopy

Do not needs?

1. ______________________________
Example: Health insurance (Spouse's employer covers it.)

2. ______________________________
Example: An active collaborator, as have 20 years experience

List your needs in order of priority.

Situation A, continued: Group of PNPs

Dr. Black wants the NPs to negotiate as a group, so that one contract fits all. However, each of the nurse practitioners has different concerns. NP Flowers, the most experienced, is most worried about how the new percentage arrangement will affect her retirement account. NP Grass, who works part-time, is worried that she will make less under the new payment arrangement than under the old arrangement. NP Tree doesn't want to sign the non-competition clause in the contract, as she wants the option of working at another practice, nearby. NP Rock is not concerned in the least about the non-competition clause, because she has decided that her next job will be in another city, more than 10 miles away. And NP Stone, the newest member of the group, just needs regular daytime work hours while her children are in school. Given that and a paycheck, NP Stone will put up with most anything. NP Stone wants to sign the contract as is and get it over with.

Situation B, continued: New NP

Having never worked as an NP before, Waters has only a vague idea what makes for a good day at work. He knows that during clinical rotations, the settings where the NP spent an hour with each patient, doing complete histories and physicals, was more satisfying than the settings where NPs saw a patient every 15 minutes.

Determining what the other party wants

There is only one way to find out what the other party wants — ask. Usually, the best person to ask is the person with whom you are negotiating. Sometimes, however, it is more productive to ask that person's assistant or associates.

If the other party is a practice owner or practice administrator, it is highly probable that the other party wants one or more of the following:

- income which exceeds expenses
- relief — time off
- someone to solve a problem; i.e. women patients want a woman clinician, or the facility has gotten poor reviews on quality measures, or patients complain that they have to wait too long to see a clinician.

A prudent question to ask at a first telephone call or interview is: "Why are you hiring someone?" For example, does the employer want to:

- Increase the size of the practice?
- Handle current overflow?
- Increase billable visits?
- Have someone with specific clinical expertise in the office?
- Have someone with clinical expertise to counsel patients?
- Have someone attend to health care maintenance?
- Have someone to cover the office on his/her days off?
- Have someone to share expenses?
- Have someone open a satellite clinic?

Situation A, continued: Group of NPs

From the language and tone of the contract Dr. Black presented the NPs, they have determined that he wants them to increase their generation of revenues, either by seeing more patients or by improving their skill at coding the visits and procedures they perform. He also wants to reduce expenses, they think, because under the new contract, expenses will be deducted from their income.

Situation B, continued: Endocrinologist wants to hire NP.

When NP Waters goes for an interview with the endocrinologist, he discovers that Dr. White is most interested in starting office hours at 10 a.m. and having Thursdays off. Dr. White wants office coverage from 8:30 a.m. to 10 a.m. and all day Thursday. Dr. White is not sure she can afford a full-time NP and would like to start with 8:30 to noon every weekday but Thursday, and 8:30 to 4:30 Thursdays. Furthermore, Dr. White is interested in having the NP do the extensive patient teaching necessary for patients with diabetes and other endocrinologic conditions.

Gathering financial data

Next, gather basic information on how the practice, agency or institution gets revenue. For example, does the practice bill insurers? If so, which insurers are the major payers? If the employer is a hospital, where does the money to support the nurse practitioner's salary come from — grants, billings to insurers, or Hill-Burton funds? If the NP's salary comes from billings to insurers, are those billings based on prospective payments for diagnostic related groups, global fees for surgery, or fees for services for evaluation and management or other procedures?

If the employer is a medical practice, gather the following data from the employer:

- What is the most frequently billed CPT code for the practice? What amount does the practice bill and receive, on average, for that CPT code?
- What percentage of practice income goes to cover practice expenses? If the employer will not reveal that information, ask how many providers share practice overhead expenses. Surveys of medical practices have shown that a solo practitioner pays 40 to 45% of income for office expenses, whereas a practice of 10 to 24 doctors pays about 20 to 25% of income for office expenses. Determine the appropriate rate to deduct for practice expenses.

3. What is the collections rate for the practice? The collections rate is the collected revenues divided by total billings, and is an indicator of the skill with which the practice files clean bills and deals with denials. A collections rate of 90% is good. A collections rate of 50% is terrible.

Situation A, continued: Group of NPs

The NPs asked Dr. Black for printouts showing billings and collections for the previous year, for each NP.

Situation B, continued: Endocrinologist wants to hire NP

NP Waters asks Dr. White for her fee schedule for Dr. White's most commonly billed CPT codes, for Medicare and for the 3 commercial payers most prevalent among Dr. White's patients.

Determine what you have to offer

Because negotiation is give and take, be prepared to state what you have to give. First, what non-monetary assets can you bring?

- Patients?
- Coverage while another clinician takes time off?
- Counseling skills?
- Help with telephone inquirics and refill requests?
- Management skills?
- Clinical expertise the other clinicians do not have?
- Style other clinicians do not have?

Second, what amount of revenue can you generate?

Income minus expenses equals profit. So, you must look at both income and expenses to determine your profitability.

Income

How much money do you bring in? Look at:

- Billable patient visits
- Procedures
- Contracts
- Capitated payments
- Grants
- Consultant fees

If you are currently employed with a practice, the billing manager may be able to supply you with the amount of your billings and collections per month, quarter or year. If the practice is unable or unwilling to provide you with that information, you may track productivity, yourself, using a notebook or a software program such as NP Data Tracker (available from Shepherd Enterprises LLC, 3 Green Valley Run, Milton, DE 19968-9317, telephone 302-645-9479, fax 302-645-4006. http://shepherdent.com/DataTrackTestimony.htm).

Consider the following regarding revenue generation:

- What do I bring to my current practice in revenues?

☐ I already know what I bring in revenues and it is
$ ________ per year.

☐ I don't know what I bring but I can find out from
________________.

☐ I don't know what I bring but I can estimate the figure by keeping track of the CPT codes I bill for a week or month, finding out the average payment for those CPT codes and calculating a yearly sum.

☐ Generation of revenues is not relevant to my situation, as I work for a non-billing government agency. However, I know where the money to support my paycheck comes from.

Situation A, continued: Group of NPs

NP Flowers, the most experienced NP in Black's group, bills $350,000 per year in fee-for-service, of which 90%, or $315,000 is collected by Dr. Black. NP Stone, the least experienced NP in the group, bills $210,000, of which 89%, or $186,900 is collected.

NP Flowers has approximately 3,000 patients who call NP Flowers "my nurse practitioner." And, NP Flowers gets lots of new patients by word of mouth from the established patients. In contrast, NP Stone tends to see Dr. Black's overflow. The other 3 NPs are somewhere between NP Flowers and NP Stone in collections and volume of patients they bring to the practice.

Situation B, continued: New NP

NP Waters has no figures to offer as proof of productivity, However, his previous work as an RN was with patients recovering from cardiac surgery. NP Waters is good at drawing blood, reading electrocardiograms, recognizing arrhythmias, performing cardiac exams and recognizing congestive heart failure. NP Waters believes he may be able to offer Dr. White something Dr. White doesn't have — this expertise in cardiac evaluation. NP Waters knows he will have to devote much of his free time during his first year in practice to studying endocrinology, if he takes this job.

Expenses

To figure expenses, answer the following questions:

- How many examination rooms do you need?
  ____
- How large an examination room do you need?
  ____________ square feet
- What is the price per square foot for office space in your area? $________

To get a rough idea of the price, consult the classified advertisements of the local newspaper, under "Professional office space."

- Do you need a separate office? ☐ Yes ☐ No
  How large?_____ square feet
- Do you need a conference room? ☐ Yes ☐ No
  How large?_____ square feet
- Do you need a reception area separate from the general reception area? ☐ Yes ☐ No
  If so, how large? _____ square feet

- How many helpers do you need?

RN ___

LPN ___

MD ___

Technician ___

Medical assistant ___

No formal training ___

- What is the yearly salary of the helpers?

RN $________

LPN $________

MD $________

Technician $________

Medical assistant $________

No formal training $________

- What salary do you want?
  $__________ per year

- What salary do you need?
  $__________ per year

- What benefits do you want?

☐ Medical insurance

☐ Dental insurance

☐ Short-term disability insurance

☐ Long-term disability insurance

☐ Retirement plan

☐ Paid vacation of ___ weeks per year

☐ Paid sick time of ___ days per year

☐ Paid personal time of ____ days per year

- What benefits do you need?

☐ Medical insurance

☐ Dental insurance

☐ Short-term disability insurance

☐ Long-term disability insurance

☐ Retirement plan

☐ Paid vacation of ___ weeks per year

☐ Paid sick time of ___ days per year

☐ Paid personal time of ____ days per year

- What practice expenses do you want the employer to pay for?

☐ Paid time off for continuing education of ____ days per year.

☐ Expenses of continuing education.

☐ Professional subscriptions to ________________, ________________.

☐ Professional dues for ________________, ________________.

☐ Professional liability insurance

☐ Hospital privileges application

☐ DEA license fees, state and federal

☐ Mobile telephone

☐ Beeper

☐ Equipment: ____________________________
(Example: Portable digital assistant with Epocrates)

☐ Uniform: ____________________________
(Example: Lab coat)

☐ Relocation expenses

☐ Advertisements regarding association with the practice, in

____

(Example: Yellow pages, local newspaper)

Expenses allocated to NP:

Salaries ________

Self ________

Helpers ________

Consulting MD ________

To calculate a reasonable salary for yourself, follow the directions in Appendix C. To determine appropriate salary for helpers, consult the local paper's classified advertisements for the type of helper you want. The rates for physician consultations run from nothing to $400 per hour. Considering that physicians can make $150 to $250 per hour seeing patients, it is probably reasonable to set the rate within that range.

Benefits

Self ________

Helpers ________

Consulting MD ________

Employees may have varying benefits. Generally, count on 25-30% of salary, depending on the number and expense of the benefits (health insurance, sick leave, vacation time, disability insurance, retirement, and so on).

Expenses of practice

Taxes ________

(8% of salary for employer's contribution to social security, Medicare)

Rent *Add the square feet of space needed and multiply by the going rate per square foot.*	________
Utilities *Estimate, for telephone, heat, electricity*	________
Malpractice Insurance	________
Continuing education classes	________
Beeper/Call Service	________
Subscriptions	________
Books	________
Professional memberships	________
Application for hospital privileges, fee	________
Supplies	________
Equipment	________
Maintenance	________
Government fees; i.e. CLIA	________
Attorney fees	________
IPA memberships	________
Approximate total expense of NP practice	________

Compare income with expenses:

Income generated by NP $__________

Expenses attributable to NP $__________

If you have administrative responsibilities, list those, and project the dollar worth of those services to the practice. Note that practice administrators are making $50,000 and up per year. Contrast the revenues brought in by the NP with the expenses attributable to the NP.

An NP prepared with print-outs of quarterly and yearly collections, estimates of practice expenses attributable to the NP, and an estimate of profits to be generated by the NP will be in a secure negotiating position with a private practice.

If an NP is applying for a job with a government agency, then it will be useful to come with the following data, if supportive of the NP:

- Attendance: Number of days missed per year, for the past 3 years
- Evaluations or letters of recommendation or commendation from previous employers
- Certifications in addition to basic certification as an NP
- Certificates of continuing education or competency in specific clinical or administrative subjects or skills

New NPs

New NPs will not have data on their actual productivity, but can project the amount of income he or she expects to generate in the first year. First, assess your speed and comfort level:

- How many patients can I see per hour, day, month, and year?

_________ per hour

_________ per day

_________ per month

_________ per year

Patient volume varies greatly among NPs, according to survey data and personal communications.

- How much physician consultation time will I need; i.e., 10-minute consultation on every patient, 5-minute consultation once a day, or 5-minute consultation once a year?

_________ minutes per day

_________ hours per week

_________ hours per month

_________ hours per year

_________ minutes per patient

New NPs often need a 5-minute consultation from an on-site collaborator after every patient visit, whereas an experienced NP may never need an on-site consultation.

- New NPs can use survey data to suggest a reasonable starting salary. A survey published in 2004 reported that the average NP salary was approximately $69,200 per year.

Marketing and other considerations

Productivity depends on an NP's speed at patient visits and procedures, and skill at billing, coding, generating business, and marketing the practice and the NP's services. To assess your readiness to negotiate, answer "Yes" or "No" to the following statements, and/or fill in the blanks:

- I have identified my "unique selling proposition" targeted at patients. ☐ Yes ☐ No

A "unique selling proposition" (USP) is a marketing term. A USP is a reason for someone to purchase what you have to offer. For example, Polly Busby, an ob-gyn nurse practitioner in Maui, Hawaii, specializes in making women patients comfortable with the annual gynecologic exam. Her advice was featured in the March 2000 issue of *Glamour Magazine*. Busby's USP is something like "I'll ease your fear or embarrassment." Other USPs for NPs might be: "Specialist in enuresis," "Specialist in wound care," "I spend the time you need," or "I concentrate on keeping you healthy."

- I have identified my USP targeted at my employer. ☐ Yes ☐ No

Hospitals, agencies and practice owners tend to be interested in four things: making money, providing coverage, solving problems, and keeping quality auditors satisfied. If an NP's worth to a practice lies in providing coverage, then the NP who provides the most coverage; i.e. is dependably present, pleasant, functional and efficient during the office hours, is the most valuable. If an NP's worth to an employer is in generating profits, then the NP's speed at procedures and skill at coding will be the NP's selling point. If the employer is most interested in demonstrating high quality of care in a nursing home, then knowledge of Minimum Data Set is a selling point. Many employers will want all 4 things — profit-generation, coverage, problem-solving and maintenance of quality. The NP who can do all of these things is practically indispensable.

- My "unique selling proposition" for my current employer is:________________________
- I am a skilled coder ☐ Yes ☐ No
- I know the differences between the levels of CPT codes relevant to my practice. ☐ Yes ☐ No
- The difference is

  Level 2 visit requires __ elements of history, __ elements of exam and ________ -level medical decision-making.

  Level 3 visit requires __ elements of history, __ elements of exam and ________ -level medical decision-making.

  For training on billing and coding evaluation and management services, see "Safe, smart billing and coding," an educational module on compact disc, available from the Law Office of Carolyn Buppert.

- I have chosen at least one measure of effectiveness in my practice and am collecting data on my effectiveness. ☐ Yes ☐ No

  Examples:

Measure: Blood pressure below 140/70.

Data: I know what percentage of my patients diagnosed with hypertension are controlled to below 140/70.

Measure: Children immunized by age 2

Data: I know the percentage of children under my care whose 2-year-old immunizations are complete.

- My example measure:

  ____

- The data I have:

  ____

For more about demonstrating effectiveness, see Buppert, C. (2000, January). Measuring outcomes in primary care practice, *Nurse Practitioner 25* (1), pp. 88-98 or Chapters 1 to 4 of Buppert, C. *The Primary Care Provider's Guide to Compensation and Quality*, Jones & Bartlett Publishers.

Summary

- I can name 2 non-monetary contributions I bring to the practice.

a) ____________________________ Example: Teach residents how to perform gynecologic examinations.

b) ______________________________ Example: Train new medical assistants.

- The monetary values I put on my non-monetary contributions are:

a) $_____ is the value of

__________________________________.

b) $_____ is the value of

__________________________________.

- Of the following "wants" common to hospitals, agencies and practice owners, I am best able to:

☐ provide services to established patients during office hours; i.e the need is for clinicians available for specified time periods

☐ provide after-hours on-call services as required by health plans

☐ assist at surgery

☐ provide a specific clinical expertise, which is

____

☐ answer patient queries or take care of problems while physicians perform procedures

☐ improve patient satisfaction

☐ take care of well women (or diabetic patients, or __________, while physicians concentrate on __________)

☐ provide a choice for patients; i.e. female provider in a predominantly male practice, or male provider in a predominantly female practice

☐ attend to preventive care and health maintenance to comply with quality standards

☐ expand the practice by bringing in new patients

☐ make money

I could bring $ __________ in profit to the practice, per year.

My prospective employer expects to make $___________ in profit from my work. Expectations for profit will vary greatly. If an employer will not tell a nurse practitioner what he or she expects in the way of profit, the nurse practitioner can insert a figure which the nurse practitioner thinks appropriate, for the purpose of negotiations.

Analyzing the fit

Given your answers to the self-assessment questions above and in the Appendices, fill in the following blanks about the means to achieve your goals:

My top 3 "wants" in a work situation are:

1.______________________________

2. ______________________________

3. ______________________________

This employer wants:

1.______________________________

2. ______________________________

3. ______________________________

The top 3 things I offer are:

1. ______________________________

2. ______________________________

3. ______________________________

The employer is most likely to be willing to give me the following of my wants:

____

The employer is least likely to be willing to give me the following of my wants:

____

I could give up ______________________.

I could not give up ______________________.

I could offer to give ______________________ in return for __________________.

Presenting wants and needs

It is probably best to present wants and needs after inquiring about the employer's wants and needs. The NP need not explain why he or she needs or wants any specific term of employment. Rather, the NP should be ready to articulate why he or she deserves a particular term or condition.

Salary

If an NP has determined that he or she needs to make $70,000 per year in order to cover a mortgage, the NP need only state "I've calculated that I need to make at least $70,000 a year." Or, "My expectation is a salary of $70,000 a year." It is not particularly relevant what the NP made at his or her last job, though an employer is likely to ask what the NP has made in the past, to gauge where the NP's salary request falls in relation to what other employers are paying. If asked, the NP may answer the question, or say something like "What I made in the past isn't relevant to me now; as I've calculated that I need to make this amount from this point forward. I'll be happy to go over my productivity numbers to demonstrate why I think my salary is justified." A new NP may say "I have made some projections of what I can bring to the practice. I think these projections show that I will bring in enough revenue to support the salary amount."

If, after an NP states his or her salary need and presents the revenue projections, the prospective employer says "The most I can offer you is $10,000 less than that," an appropriate response is to pause just a moment, then state, matter of factly, "That just won't do" (if that is the case). Say nothing more about the matter until the employer responds. If there is no response after about 10 seconds, thank the individual for the interview and exit.

Negotiating with a practice owner can be easier, or more difficult, than negotiating with a hospital administrator. A practice owner will see an NP's salary as a reduction in the amount the owner can draw from the practice, rather than as a line item in a budget. The practice owner knows that he or she either has more money but less time than he or she needs, or that he or she needs the money. While the practice owner can make quick decisions, he or she may be emotionally attached to the dollars paid to an NP. A hospital administrator, on the other hand, is negotiating with someone else's money. The hospital may have a salary range, within which the administrator may negotiate. If the hospital has a cap on the salary that can be offered an NP, getting more may mean getting corporate executive approval.

No matter who the NP is negotiating with, if there are several qualified candidates, the candidate who will accept $55,000 may get the job, instead of the candidate who holds out for $70,000. On the other hand, if there are few candidates, or the candidate who wants $70,000 is clearly a better fit than any other candidate, the hospital administrator or practice owner may give the higher-priced NP what he or she wants.

It is appropriate for a candidate for a job to ask whether there are other applicants, and where the candidate stands in relation to those applicants.

Non-monetary terms and conditions

Often, an NP's needs include working conditions which are not directly related to money. For example, an NP may need to finish work every day at 3 p.m. in order to pick up children at school or attend class. Or, the NP may be active in a professional or community organization, and may need certain days off throughout the year. If so, the NP should simply state the need. The NP need not state the reason behind the need.

Details for a working relationship may or may not be covered in an employment agreement. If a NP wants specific terms, it is appropriate to state that at the second interview. The categories of terms commonly seen in employment agreements for NPs are:

- Clinical duties
- Administrative duties
- Committee work
- Performance measurement
- Responsibility for promoting the practice
- Scope of practice
- Hours/sessions/appointment slots
- Assistance/Assistants
- Practice sites and settings
- Terms of on-call services
- Conditions for termination
- Terms of non-competition
- Safety and standard of care
- Compensation: Salary and bonuses
- Practice expenses to be paid
- Benefits
- Billing on behalf of NP
- Stipulations regarding outside work
- Ownership of patient charts, mailing lists
- Term of agreement

To elicit information from the prospective employer, ask such questions as:

- Is call required? If so, how is call shared? What back-up will I have if consultation is needed for a call?
- What kind of support staff will the practice provide?
- How many support staff will the practice provide?

- What will support staff do for me? What will support staff expect me to do for them?
- To whom will I report? About medical issues? About administrative issues? About payment issues?
- What quality improvement methods does the practice use?
- If I have wanted to organize my daily practice routine, and the routine is different from the current process, could I change the current process?
- Am I expected to build a panel of patients, or cover for overbookings of the other providers, or both?

Be prepared to answer the following questions:

- Why should I hire an NP?
- Why should I hire you?
- How many patients are you used to seeing in a day?
- Do you have a DEA number?
- How independently are you used to practicing? How often do you need a consultation?
- What can you bring to the practice?
- What is your greatest job strength? Weakness?
- What can an NP legally do in this state?
- What do you want to be doing in 2 years? In 5 years? In 10 years?
- Are evening and/or weekend hours possible for you?

Give and take

Once the needs of both parties are understood, the bargaining can begin. There may or may not be room for give and take. For example, if an employer's reason for hiring an NP is to get coverage between 3 and 5 p.m., so that the employer may spend time with small children, and one of the NP's top priority need is to be finished with work by 3 p.m. in order to spend time with small children, then this employer and this NP will not be well matched. In this example, there may be no room for give and take. In most instances, employer or employee can propose a solution which will fit both parties' needs. For example, if an NP needs to make $70,000 a year, and the employer had planned on paying only $60,000 a year, the NP might propose a percentage of collections arrangement such that the NP is guaranteed a salary of $60,000 a year, and has the opportunity to make an extra $10,000 by conducting an evening clinic in which all collections would accrue to the NP. Or, the NP may know of a grant or contract which the NP could bring to the practice. Or, the NP may take a job with less salary than desired, in order to get experience, so that he or she can negotiate a higher salary for future job opportunities.

Dealing with distractions

There are 3 tactics which can throw and NP off balance when negotiating — the "red herring," the "I need to check" tactic, and the delay tactic.

Red herring

"Red herring" is an expression meaning "an attempt to distract attention from the real question."[1] For example, a trucking company offered an employee in the sales department a stock option, saying "We want to reward your 25 years of service with this offer of 500 shares of company stock. This is the first time we have ever honored an employee in this way. Please sign this acceptance letter in order to take advantage of this offer." The acceptance letter included a paragraph in

1 An Internet search for the derivation of the term "red herring" revealed that in the 1800s, a curing process turned herring a red color. The cured fish were particularly strong smelling. Participants in a fox hunt would sometimes tie a herring to a string and drag it through the woods to confuse the hounds, either as a test when training the dogs or as a competitive tactic. According to one web site, fugitives (in the 1800s) might rub a red herring across their trail, diverting the bloodhounds in pursuit. The term is also used in investment circles to refer to a preliminary prospectus that is incomplete and could be misleading.

which the employee agreed not to work for another trucking company in the future. This employee was nearing the age where he could retire from his present employment, and indeed planned to seek a position with another trucking company, where he could use his existing sales contacts. By offering the stock options, his current employer was hoping to divert the employee's attention from the employer's goal of getting the employee's promise not to compete in the future.

The way to deal with red herring is simply to recognize it, and not let it blind one to more important matters.

"Need to check"

If an individual you are negotiating with cannot make a decision, it is probable that the negotiations are being conducted at the wrong level of management. An NP may be wasting his or her time if the party with whom he or she is negotiating has to constantly check with someone else before making a decision. Some parties use this tactic to make the other party nervous, by suggesting that the requests are unreasonable and unusual.

The way to deal with this tactic is to ask to negotiate with the individual who has the authority to make a binding agreement.

Delay

Some parties participate in negotiations but drag their feet when it comes to making a final decision. The only way to deal with delay tactics is to say or write something like this: "My offer is good for 30 days, or until I agree to take another job, whichever comes first."

Closing

In general:

- Hold firm on your top priorities. Give in on less important terms, in return for concessions on more important terms. Expect the employer to do the same.

- Negotiate your final deal individually, rather than as part of a group of NPs.
- If you come to an impasse about a particular term, move on to other terms, or stop negotiations and take some time to reconsider.
- Evaluate other job options, so that if Plan A cannot be worked out, you will be in a position of strength by having Plan B as back-up.
- If there is a stalemate, your needs are firm, and the terms being offered do not appreciate and reward the value you bring, politely back out of the negotiations, and explain why. You can always turn around and come back if the employer becomes more flexible.

PART 3

Contract language

An employment contract is a written agreement under which the employee and employer state the terms and conditions of a working relationship. It is important that the contract language be straightforward and precise. One wants to avoid a situation where the parties are both reading the language, but one party interprets the language to mean one thing, and the other party interprets it to mean something else.

Does an NP need a written employment contract?

Many NPs have practiced for many years without employment contracts. In the past, an employer offered a salary and benefits in return for a certain number of hours per week. Other details were decided upon as issues arose, but NPs sometimes were unhappy with how the decisions were made. For example, an NP took a job that did not require on-call services. Later, the NP was told that she would be on-call 3 nights a week, without additional compensation. The NP had no legal recourse.

Contracts have certain advantages over informal employment arrangements. First, contract negotiation forces parties to discuss issues. When the parties agree on specific terms, there is a document which records the agreement, and which can be referred to as necessary to refresh memories about details of the agreement. In most cases, an employment agreement is protective to both employer and employee.

An NP who has a properly written contract is guaranteed a job for the duration of the contract. An employer who wants to end the employment of the NP would have to wait until the contract terminates, or attempt to settle the matter with the NP, possibly by offering severance terms.

Why would an employer want a contract?

An effectively written employment agreement protects an employer against competition from an employee who leaves the practice and takes patients to another practice. The method of restricting competition is a "restrictive covenant," a clause commonly seen in employment agreements for NPs, physicians, veterinarians and dentists. Examples of restrictive covenants are given later.

And, because employers bill insurers for work performed by NPs, employers want to make it clear that receivables are the property of the employer, that the NP is committed to specific sessions, and that the patients' records stay with the practice, unless the patient specifically directs otherwise.

What rights does an employed NP have, without a contract?

In most states, employment is "at will." At-will employment means the employment continues as long as both parties want to continue. If one party wants out, the arrangement ends. Without a contract for a specified term of employment, an employee has no legal right to a job. Likewise, an employee may quit employment at any time, barring a contract for a specified term. The only protections for an employee are those offered by the equal opportunity and disability laws; i.e., an employee cannot be terminated solely on the basis of age, gender, race, or disability.

An NP who is employed but has no contract may negotiate terms of employment on a piecemeal basis, relying on the ability of the NP and the other party to reach agreement as issues arise. If an employer changes the pay scale or work responsibilities for the better, the NP benefits. If the employer reduces the pay scale or unreasonably increases responsibilities, the NP has no recourse but to keep working under the new conditions, or leave.

Contract terms

Some of the issues often addressed in an employment contract are:

- scope of services to be performed
- compensation
- duration of employment
- how agreement can be altered or updated
- responsibility to maintain credentials
- terms of on-call responsibilities
- benefits
- time off and expenses for continuing education
- vacation time
- number of office hours per week
- restriction on competition
- bonuses
- reasons for termination
- assistance with continuing education

Some issues which often are not addressed, but can be dealt with in an employment contract, are:

- extent of support services — office assistants and clinical assistants — to be offered NP
- expectations regarding the number of patients seen per day
- expectations regarding non-clinical (administrative work) to be done by NP
- listing of NP on door, in directories, in advertisements
- use of NP's name when office telephone is answered
- release to NP of NP's quality performance as measured by health plan auditors

An employment agreement can include anything the parties wish to address. Often, agreements are written by attorneys for the practice, and therefore are oriented to the needs of the employer.

Three difficult clauses: Restrictive covenants, bonus formulas, and termination

Three clauses commonly found in employment agreements offered by medical practices to NPs are especially difficult for NPs to interpret, and can have profound effects on an NP's life. It is these clauses which often bring NPs to attorneys for advice. These clauses are restrictive covenants, bonus formulas, and termination clauses. Restrictive covenants require a nurse practitioner to promise — before accepting employment, or if already employed, as a condition of continued employment — not to compete with an employer when the present employment ends. Bonus formulas specify conditions under which an employer rewards an NP for superior performance. Termination clauses specify that an employer may end the agreement, without cause, with thirty days' notice.

Restrictive covenants

A restrictive covenant is a promise not to compete. Specifically, a restrictive covenant is a clause which restricts an employee from practicing in the same specialty as the employer, within a set number of miles from an employer's business, for a set period of time after the employee leaves the employer's business.

An employer wants to avoid a situation where a departing NP takes patients to the next NP position. NPs, on the other hand, want to be able to take the best job offer available. Sometimes the best job offer is geographically close to the NP's previous job. Restrictive covenants are legal and enforceable, as long as they are reasonable. "Reasonable" means different things in different contexts. A judge will determine whether or not a clause is reasonable, if the matter goes to court.

If an NP who has signed a non-compete agreement leaves an employer and joins the practice next door, the former employer may decide to take the NP to court, seeking to enforce the contract, and asking the court to issue an injunction prohibiting the employee from practicing. Sometimes, a former employee will challenge the validity of a restrictive covenant by taking the matter to court, and asking a judge will determine whether a restrictive covenant is reasonable. Before making a decision, a judge would analyze the past court decisions in the state, and then compare the facts of those cases with the current case. Such facts might be the size of the city or town where the practice is located, the severity of the geographic and time restrictions in the clause, the availability of other health care providers, and what the employment climate is like for health care providers. The judge would balance the needs of the employer against the harm to the employee. The judge would decide whether the geographic restriction and the time restriction were appropriate to accomplish the employer's needs, but no more. Finally, the judge would consider whether there is any potential injury to the public if a restrictive covenant is enforced.

Judges have found restrictive covenants unreasonable when the restriction on the former employee is greater than necessary to protect the legitimate business interests of the employer. Judges also have found restrictive covenants unreasonable when the restriction creates a hardship for the employee. Occasionally, judges have found restrictive covenants to be unreasonable when there is neither excessive restraint nor excessive hardship, but there is a likely injury to the public.

For example, a covenant restricting an oral surgeon from practicing in a particular city for 3 years after termination from a practice was found to be unreasonable. The restraint was greater than necessary, said the judge. However, a covenant restricting a veterinarian from practicing in a different city for 3 years after termination was found to be reasonable. In that case, the restraint was not greater than necessary, the judge held. In yet another case, a covenant restricting a physician from practicing in a rural town for 3 years after termination was found to be unreasonable. In that case there was a potential injury to the public. The injury to the public was a potential shortage of physicians, because the town had only 2 physicians. The difference in outcome in these 3 cases can be reconciled only by comparing the factual details of the cases. A decision that one clause was reasonable while a seemingly identical clause was unreasonable was due to differences in profession, practice, city, availability of other providers and many other factors.

When negotiating the terms of a restrictive covenant, an NP needs to consider the circumstances of the job offer, the severity of the restriction, the potential hardship imposed on the NP by the covenant, the availability of health care providers in the area, and the availability of other practice opportunities.

In agreeing to a restrictive covenant, an NP is giving up something of value — the ability to take any other NP job which is offered. However, an NP who refuses to sign a reasonable restrictive covenant may be seen by an employer as someone who is looking to start a competing practice nearby. The best advice on restrictive covenants is to negotiate one the NP can live with; i.e., one which seems reasonable for all concerned, under the particular circumstances of the practice and the NP. And, insist that the employer give the NP something of value in return for the promise to restrict opportunities for future practice.

Examples of more reasonable and less reasonable restrictive covenants are provided in Table 1.

Table 1

Restrictive covenants: Employee's promise not to compete

Example 1: "Upon termination of employment for any reason, employee agrees not to practice in any location within **25 miles of any present or future office of this practice for a period of 5 years.**"

ANALYSIS:

Accomplishes employer's need for protection, but

May be broader than necessary to accomplish employer's need, and

May put excessive hardship on employee.

Example 2: "Upon termination of employment for any reason, NP agrees not to practice in any location within **1 mile of the Jones Road office of this practice for a period of 1 year.**"

ANALYSIS:

Not a hardship on employee, but

May not accomplish employer's need for protection, as patients may be willing to travel one mile to see NP

Bonus formulas

Some employers offer NPs the opportunity for bonuses. The criteria for bonuses vary greatly from practice to practice. The most important criteria for bonuses are that both employer and employee understand the formula, and that it be ethical from the point of view of the patient.

The most common problem with bonus formulas is vague language. If a formula is vague, it may be interpreted in different ways by different individuals, and there could be disagreements and disappointments when it comes time for distribution of the bonus.

Productivity-based formulas

Many formulas are based on the number of patient visits per year, the number of relative value units billed, or the amount of revenue generated per quarter or per year. This makes good business sense under a fee-for-service system of reimbursement. If a practice is at least half fee-for-service, patient visit-based formulas can be a reasonable choice. Generally, an NP who sees large numbers of patients is a productive employee who deserves a bonus.

Bonus formulas based on numbers of patient visits make less sense when reimbursement to the practice is capitated. Under capitated reimbursement, a practice is paid a set fee per patient per month, regardless of the number of patient visits. Under capitated reimbursement, the ultimate goal is not a high number of visits from each patient, but good patient care in as few visits as possible. Though many practices use patient visit volume to determine clinicians' bonuses, even when the patients are capitated, a formula based on visits makes little sense. On the other hand, employers have to be careful not to give providers bonuses for withholding care. Under capitated reimbursement, it may make the most sense to award a bonus based on some measure of quality of care or outcome.

Many practices receive payments under both fee-for-service schedules and capitation schedules. If that is the case, it may be equitable to base bonuses on relative value units, or use a formula like the one provided in Appendix C under "For a practice with capitated patients," and then apply a percentage to the productivity number.

Quality-based bonuses

While performance measures are more difficult to track than patient visits, they are more suited to managed care. Some health plans supply performance data to practices, and this data could be used to determine bonuses.

Bonuses can be awarded when the percentage of patients who have met health maintenance standards — such as childhood immunizations complete by age 2 or mammograms performed every 2 years for women over 50 — exceeds a benchmark, such as 80% performed and documented. Or, bonuses could be awarded if emergency room visits declined in the past year.

In order to track performance data and apportion bonuses based on performance, patients and primary providers must be paired. NPs will need to have their own panels of patients, and be designated as primary care provider for that panel. Or, NP/physician teams could work together and share bonuses.

Profit-based formulas

Some employers share profits with NPs. This can be satisfying to both employer and employee, as long as the method for determining profits is clear.

NPs should be aware that there are accounting methods which can maximize or minimize profits. "Profit" is a word which has modifiers, such as "gross" and "net," which can mean the difference between a bonus and no bonus. NPs who agree to profit-based formulas should negotiate for the right to audit financial records. And, there should be a process for resolving disputes about profit calculations.

Patient satisfaction-based formulas

Patient satisfaction is subjective, difficult to measure, and open to conflicting interpretations. On the other hand, there are a multitude of patient satisfaction tools available, and if employer and employee can agree upon a method of measurement, patient satisfaction certainly can be part of a bonus formula.

Bonus formulas are controversial. Many practices are struggling with this issue. One approach being taken by employers is to implement a bonus formula with the understanding that it will be altered and fine-tuned from year to year.

See Table 2 for some examples of bonus formulas which have been offered to NPs.

Table 2

Bonus formulas

Example clause #1: Up to 15% percent of base salary, 5% if practice is profitable; 5% based on meeting a threshold of patient visits; 5% based on patient satisfaction, staff satisfaction and citizenship.

Example clause #2: The product of "collected billings" multiplied by "total employee billings" divided by "total practice billings," with a cap.

Example clause #3: A figure determined by a committee, based on meeting criteria for a) financial performance, b) quality of medical services determined by outcomes, medical appropriateness and extent of health promotion services provided, and e) level of patient satisfaction.

All of these clauses are vague. Given a specific set of facts and the parties' expectations, the wording could be clarified.

Termination without cause

Typically, the Termination section of an employment agreement will list events which are the basis for termination of the employee "for cause." These events often include conviction of a felony, loss of license, loss of hospital privileges, and gross negligence which compromises patient safety.

In addition to "termination for cause" provisions, some employment agreements include a "termination without cause" clause, which states that employer can terminate employee at any time, without cause, with 30 days' notice. See examples, Table 3, "Termination clauses."

A termination without cause clause defeats the purpose of a contract for an employee. An employee who can be terminated at any time for any reason, or for no reason, not only has no job security but will think twice about pressing for performance of any of the other provisions in the employment agreement. For example, an NP may believe a bonus was due, while the employer believes no bonus was due. If the NP protests too much, an employer can simply terminate the NP. If, on the other hand, an NP can be terminated only "for cause," then the NP will feel freer to be assertive about the other provisions of the contract.

There are reasons to agree to a "termination without cause" clause, however. If an NP cannot commit to a full year's employment, it may be best to agree to the "without cause" clause. Most employers will not agree to delete a "without cause" clause unless the employee also gives up the right to leave with just 30 days notice.

Table 3

Termination clauses

Example: Termination for cause clause

> Employer may terminate this agreement at the sole discretion of employer, by written notice to the NP upon the occurrence of any of the following:
>
> a) The NP dies or becomes disabled....
>
> b) The NP loses his or her professional license....
>
> c) The NP is limited or restricted by any governmental authority having jurisdiction over the NP to the extent that the NP cannot render the required professional services....

Example for Table 3: Termination without cause clause (Not recommended)

The employer may terminate this agreement at any time, for any reason, after 30 days' notice to NP.

A check list

Use the following checklist to determine whether you have addressed all of the issues:

Scope of services

☐ Is after-hours call required?

☐ Will the NP be conducting hospital visits? Nursing home visits? Visits on weekends and evenings? Visits at satellite clinics?

☐ Are administrative duties expected of the NP?

Duration of the employment arrangement

☐ Is the term of employment stated? What is it?

Compensation

☐ Is it clear what salary is agreed upon?

Benefits:

☐ Health plan premiums

☐ Retirement plan contribution

☐ Continuing education tuition and expenses paid

☐ Professional liability insurance paid

☐ Professional dues paid

☐ DEA license fees

☐ Hospital admission privilege fee

☐ Vacation

☐ License fees paid

- ☐ Life insurance
- ☐ Disability insurance
- ☐ Holidays
- ☐ Sick time
- ☐ Bereavement leave
- ☐ Automobile mileage
- ☐ Cell phone
- ☐ Beeper

Staff support to be provided by practice

- ☐ How many assistants?
- ☐ Front office receptionist?
- ☐ Lab technician?
- ☐ Assistant for follow-up of diagnostic test results?

Restriction on other professional activities

- ☐ Is NP free to consult elsewhere?
- ☐ Is NP free to practice elsewhere?

Termination

- ☐ Are circumstances clearly stated under which the contract may be terminated prior to the end of the stated term of the contract?

Non-competition

- ☐ Must the NP agree to limit his/her activities after leaving employment?
- ☐ If so, are the limits unreasonable?

Bonus

☐ Is there opportunity for a bonus?

☐ Is the language describing the opportunity clear?

☐ Is there a means by which a disagreement between employee and employer over the amount of bonus due could be resolved?

Getting legal advice

While the negotiating is best done by the parties to the contract, contract review is best done by an attorney. An attorney who is familiar with contracts, business issues, medical practice issues and nurse practitioners is a good first choice. A logical second choice would be an attorney who reviews contracts of other health care providers — physicians, in particular.

Avoid the attorney who needs to research the law regarding NPs. One NP spent $1500 for an attorney to research the law on NPs, only to find that she knew the answers to the questions he was looking up.

Attorneys charge between $75 and $400 an hour. Many will negotiate a flat fee for reviewing a contract. It is worth spending $400 (though not $400 an hour) for review of a contract that is worth between $70,000 and $100,000 per year to the NP. If an attorney finds vague wording which needs to be made more specific, the investment in the attorney will be repaid in the long run.

What to do if contract terms are not honored

If, after a contract is signed and the parties have been working together for a period of time, a nurse practitioner finds that he or she is asked to do something that is not covered by the contract, or the employer fails to provide some benefit specified by the contract, the NP should do the following:

1. Bring up the subject orally, in private.

2. State what the NP wants.

3. Have the contract in hand.

4. Ask for a commitment; for example, the problem will be resolved within a time frame.

5. If the deadline passes, and the contract is still not being honored, follow up with a letter, restating what the NP wants and requesting a response by a stated date.

6. If still no resolution, the NP has 3 choices — live with it, leave, or file suit in state court for "specific performance."

Making revisions

It is common to want to change some part of an existing contract without renegotiating and rewriting the entire contract. A change may be made by writing an addendum, of any length, which refers to a specific paragraph and states the addition, deletion or change to be made in the contract. Both parties must sign the addendum. The addendum should state that the portions of the contract not covered by the addendum will remain in effect.

A few final points

Few people find it easy to negotiate for themselves. That is why professional athletes, authors and performers have agents. Agents, however, cost money and have their own contract issues to negotiate. Nurse practitioners can negotiate their own working terms and conditions. Even when the job market is tight, a nurse practitioner's services and expertise are valuable, and the nurse practitioner deserves respectable terms of employment.

In some situations, however, a nurse practitioner will want to simply agree to whatever terms the employer wants, assuming that the arrangement is legal and does not put the nurse practitioner at risk for loss of license or malpractice. For example, a nurse practitioner may want to get experience in a new specialty or may need to move quickly to a new town where the nurse practitioner has no contacts. The bottom line for the nurse practitioner may be "I want this job, even if I don't get to check off the items in my priority list." In that case, take the job and begin preparations for negotiations next year for a better package.

For most nurse practitioners, the most valuable piece of advice regarding negotiations is one word: "Ask."

Appendix A—Auditing the Current Job

Self-audit statement:

1. My job enables me to develop specific expertise.
   ☐ Yes ☐ No

2. My job enables me to become recognized in some way for my expertise. ☐ Yes ☐ No

3. I know exactly what my services are worth; i.e. I can identify 3 services I provide and can state the fee that comes into the practice or facility from my provision of those services. ☐ Yes ☐ No

4. My opinion counts when policy decisions are made.
   ☐ Yes ☐ No

5. My employer is aware of the language of the Nurse Practice Act in my state. ☐ Yes ☐ No

6. I am practicing within the scope of practice for a nurse practitioner, as stated in the Nurse Practice Act in my state. ☐ Yes ☐ No

7. If there is any service I am providing that is not clearly within the scope of practice for a nurse practitioner in my state, I have been delegated the authority to provide that service, by a physician, in writing.
   ☐ Yes ☐ No

8. There are systems in the facility or practice where I work which ensure that the results of diagnostic tests I order are received, and abnormal tests are followed up.
   ☐ Yes ☐ No

9. If I am off one day, or sick, and an abnormal test result comes back, someone else in the practice or facility will be

notified and will be responsible for follow up as needed.
☐ Yes ☐ No

10. I understand the method by which my job performance is evaluated. ☐ Yes ☐ No

11. Day to day, I understand what my employer expects of me. ☐ Yes ☐ No

12. I am confident that my facility or practice strives to practice ethically and legally. ☐ Yes ☐ No

13. I prescribe only those medications which I believe are medically necessary and beneficial to a patient — I'm not pressured to refill questionable prescriptions written by other clinicians at my practice. ☐ Yes ☐ No

14. My coworkers and I are reasonably compatible regarding what we want to accomplish. ☐ Yes ☐ No

15. My coworkers, in general, are pleasant. ☐ Yes ☐ No

16. I feel physically safe at work. ☐ Yes ☐ No

17. I can advance professionally in this job — through promotion, opportunity to make more money, or opportunity to be involved in satisfying projects. ☐ Yes ☐ No

18. The level of responsibility my job/employer demands is reasonably related to my salary; i.e. low salary and low responsibility or high salary and high responsibility.
☐ Yes ☐ No

19. I have the authority, within the practice or corporate structure, to make the decisions that need to be made to do my job well. ☐ Yes ☐ No

20. I feel that my employer values my contribution to the practice, facility or company. ☐ Yes ☐ No

If the percentage of "Yes" answers (number of "Yes" answers divided by the total number of answers) is less than 70%, look for other opportunities or request that specific changes take place in the working conditions, with changes completed within 6 months.

APPENDIX B—A SELF-ASSESSMENT OF "WANTS"

The following self-assessment questions may be helpful:

1. I know what makes my day, and it is:____.

2. It is most important to me to (rank in order of importance)

   - ☐ Work as part of a team
   - ☐ Feel connected to my coworkers
   - ☐ Feel like I am a standout among my peers
   - ☐ Feel indispensable to my patients
   - ☐ Be able to make a certain level of income, which is $ ________________
   - ☐ Take on and be successful at new challenges
   - ☐ Have a place to go every day
   - ☐ Have health insurance for my family
   - ☐ Have sufficient time off to pursue other interests
   - ☐ Make my own work plans and carry them out
   - ☐ Have a high level of control over my working environment

3. The type of job I would really like involves (rank in order of importance):

   - ☐ Control over my paycheck; i.e. the more work I do the more I get paid
   - ☐ A dependable paycheck
   - ☐ Lots of time off

- ☐ My having control over when and how I do my work
- ☐ New and different challenges most all of the time
- ☐ My carrying out other people's designs, orders and plans
- ☐ A specific expertise of mine
- ☐ Exposure to interesting people
- ☐ Connecting me to my community

Appendix C—Calculating reasonable salary

An NP's salary will depend on:

- What the NP has to offer
- How well the NP negotiates
- Whether or not the NP is willing to work fast and long for a productivity-based salary
- The cost of the NP's benefits
- How badly an employer wants to hire an NP
- The profit an employer is expecting to make
- How many other nurse practitioners want the job
- The salary other nurse practitioners are willing to take
- Whether or not physicians are competing for the same job, and if so, the salary these physicians are willing to take

There are 4 methods of payment currently being used to pay employed NPs.

- Straight salary
- Percentage of net receipts
- Base salary plus percentage
- Hourly rate

In a straight salary arrangement, a NP is paid a set amount to perform according to a job description. In a percentage salary arrangement, a NP is paid the amount the NP bills minus accounts receivable, minus the NP's portion of practice expenses (which includes the expense of physician consultation). In a base salary plus percentage arrangement, a NP is guaranteed a set salary, but can make additional salary if the NP generates practice income over some set amount. NPs working on an hourly basis are paid only for the hours worked.

Straight salary and hourly are more commonly encountered arrangements than percentage or set salary plus percentage.

The advantage of percentage-based salaries is the opportunity for productive NPs to have some control over their earnings. The disadvantage is that the method sets up fellow providers in a practice as competitors for patients.

No matter what arrangement an NP chooses, it is wise to focus on hard figures which document an NP's monetary contribution to a practice, and the costs of an NP to a practice.

NPs bring in income on a fee-for-service basis or a per-member-per-month basis. Figuring an NP's share of income for a fee-for-service practice is done by multiplying the number of visits by the collected fee per visit. When a practice's patients are capitated, an NP's share of income is figured by multiplying the number of patients on an NP's panel by the per-member-per-month fee coming into the practice.

To calculate whether your salary expectations are realistic:

For an office-based, fee-for-service practice:

A. How much do you want to make in salary per year?

____

B. How many patients do you want to see per day?

____

C. Are there enough patients in your practice for you to book your schedule as full as you would like?

____

D. How many days a week will you work?

____

E. How many weeks vacation do you require?

____

F. How many days of sick leave do you need per year?

____

G. How many holidays will you take?

____

H. How many days will you need for CME?

____

I. Based on answers for D-H, how many weeks per year will you work? ____________

J. How many patients will you see per year?
Multiply days/week (D) x weeks/year (I)
x patients/day (B)

____

K. What is the most common CPT code you bill?

____

Multiply: Patients/year (J) x the physician's fee for that code
minus any discounts
minus any reduction applied to NPs =

____

Approximate $ productivity

For a practice with capitated patients:

If the NP has patients specifically assigned to the NP:

1. Identify the patients under the NP's care.
2. Determine the cap rate for the patients.
3. Total the monthly income from the patients under the NP's care. Annualize the figure.

If the NP shares responsibility with other providers in the practice:

1. Determine the number of visits to the NP from capitated patients. (Example: NP saw 1,000 HMO patients last year.)
2. Determine the number of visits to the group from capitated patients. (Example: Group saw 10,000 HMO patients last year.)

3. Determine income to the group through capitation. (Example: Capitation income equals $500,000/year.)

4. Divide group's income from capitation by the number of visits to the group from patients covered by capitation. This will give you a per-visit charge. (Example: $500,000 ÷ 10,000= $50/patient visit)

5. Multiply the per-visit charge by the number of visits conducted by the NP. This will be the productivity figure for the NP for capitated patients. (Example: $50 x 1,000 = $50,000).

To project an appropriate salary for a particular NP:

1) calculate income to the practice based on NP billings

2) subtract 10% for unpaid bills

3) subtract

a) the calculated figure for practice expenses (20 to 50% of earnings)

b) the cost of physician consultation (10 to 20% of net earnings), and

c) a percentage for employer profit

Fee-for-service practices

For example, an NP who sees 15 patients per day at $35 per patient visit, on average, brings in $525 per day. Allowing for one week off for continuing education, one week off for illness, and 4 weeks off for vacation, this NP will bring in $120,750 a year, potentially.[2] But not all bills are paid. With a 90% collections rate—a reasonable collection rate for an efficient practice—this NP actually will bring in $108,675 per year.

An NP who sees 24 patients per day will bring in $840 per day, or $193,200 per year in accounts receivable. With a 90% collections rate, this NP will bring $173,880 to the practice.

2 Amount of vacation, sick or personal leave taken, varying fee schedules and other factors will affect billings and collections.

Deducting 40% of the NP's gross generated income for overhead expenses (rent, benefits, continuing education, supplies, malpractice, lab expenses, and depreciation of equipment), leaves $65,205 for the 15-patient-per-day NP and $104,328 for the 24-patient-per-day NP.

Further deducting 15% of that figure to pay a physician for consultation services leaves $55,425 in salary for the 15-patient-per-day NP and $88,679 in salary for the 24-patient-per-day NP.

Deducting 10% for employer profit leaves $49,882 in salary for the 15-patient-per-day NP and $79,811 for the 24-patient-per-day NP.

Capitated practices

In a fully-capitated practice, an NP who has a panel of 1,000 patients at an average fee per-member-per-month of $10 will bring in $120,000 annually. There should be a 100% collection rate under a capitated system of reimbursement.

Applying 40% to overhead leaves $72,000, and paying 15% (of $72,000) for physician consultation and 10% (of the remaining $61,200) for employer profit leaves $55,080 for NP salary.[3] An NP with a larger panel will make more.

The new NP

A newly graduated NP without experience may be able to see only 10 patients a day, with frequent 5- to 10-minute physician consultations per day, for the first 6 months. Plugging in the figures as in the examples above, the NP will bill 2,400 visits per year (2 weeks vacation for the new grad) at $35 per visit to total $84,000 in accounts receivable. With a 90% collection rate, the new NP will bring in $75,600.

Deduct 40% for practice expenses, which brings the net income to $45,360.

Because a new NP often requires significant consultation time

---

3 Calculations could be done differently. For example, the 10% for employer profit could be taken from the difference between collections and overhead; in this case, $72,000.

with a physician (or experienced NP), deduct 25% ($11,340) for payment for consultation, bringing the NP salary down to $34,020. With a 10% contribution to employer profit, this new NP's appropriate salary is down to $30,618.

After 6 months, when the same NP becomes more comfortable and more efficient, the income numbers should double, and consultation requirements should decrease, so that the appropriate salary would more closely approximate the salary of the 15-patient-per-day NP, and, eventually the 24-patient-per-day NP, used in the examples above. Many employers start a new NP at a salary significantly higher than $30,618, expecting that low productivity in the first 6 months will be balanced by high productivity in the second half of the year.

The experienced NP

Experienced NPs who are seeing more than 15 patients per day at CPT code level 99213 or higher should be making least $50,000 per year. If not, there are inefficiencies in the practice, or an NP is not sharing in his or her profits.

Are these projections accurate?

One could argue about whether the percentages used above are correct. In fact, some practices have poor rates of collections, some practices have higher overhead expenses, some physicians want more payment for consultation than $9,780 per year for a 15-patient-per-day NP or $15,649 per year for a 24-patient-per-day NP, and some employers want more profit than projected here. However, a nurse practitioner should not be subsidizing a poorly run practice and should not be overcompensating a physician or employer.

A template employment contract, suitable for a nurse practitioner contracting to work in an office practice, is available for purchase from Law Office of Carolyn Buppert. The contract is on disk, is available in Word or Word Perfect, and comes with instructions. Price is $250.

Order Form

SHIP TO:

PURCHASER/LICENSEE NAME

ADDRESS

PRODUCT	PRICE	QTY	TOTAL
Negotiating for Nurse Practitioners (book)	$35 each		
Avoiding Malpractice: 10 rules, 5 systems, 20 cases (book)	$35 each		
The Green Sheet: The latest on compensation and reimbursement for NPs (monthly newsletter)	$35 per year		
The Gold Sheet: The latest on quality for NPs (monthly newsletter)	$35 per year		
Safe, smart billing and coding for evaluation and management (training modules on compact disk) (See www. buppert.com for description and additional pricing structures.)	$99 PER INDIVIDUAL LICENSEE. $600 FOR LICENSE FOR UNIVERSITY PROGRAM		
Template employment contract (13 pages, with 12 pages of instructions) ☐in Word 6.0 for Windows ☐in Word Perfect 6.0	$250 each		
Billing Physician Services Provided by Nurse Practitioners in Specialist's offices, Hospitals, Nursing facilities, Homes and Hospices (book)	$89 each		
		Maryland residents must include 5% sales tax	
		TOTAL	

To order Buppert's books published by Jones & Bartlett, call 1-800-852-0034, extension 8197

SHIPPING IS INCLUDED

PAYMENT INFORMATION:

☐ Check or Money Order (Payable to Law Office of Carolyn Buppert)

For additional information, visit **www.buppert.com** or call (443) 482-3360

Please allow up to 2 weeks for US delivery. Prices are subject to change without notice.

About the Author

Carolyn Buppert is an attorney and nurse practitioner who specializes in the legal issues affecting medical practices and nurse practitioners.

She is the author of 4 other books and an instructional module on compact disk. The books are *The Nurse Practitioner's Business Practice and Legal Guide* (2004, Jones & Bartlett Publishers), *The Primary Care Provider's Guide to Compensation and Quality* (2004, Jones & Bartlett Publishers), *Avoiding Malpractice* (2004, Law Office of Carolyn Buppert), and *Billing Physician Services Provided by Nurse Practitioners in Specialist's offices, Hospitals, Nursing facilities, Homes and Hospices* (2004, Law Office of Carolyn Bupert). The instructional module is *Safe, smart billing and coding: Evaluation and Management* (2004, Law Office of Carolyn Buppert).

Ms. Buppert is a frequent contributor to various nursing publications. Her articles appear on Medscape.com, and she is on Medscape's nursing editorial board. She lectures extensively on avoiding malpractice, reimbursement issues, and negotiating contracts. Her web site, which includes links to many of her articles, is www.buppert.com.

In 2000, *The Nurse Practitioner* (a journal) named her Nurse Practitioner of the Year.

CONTACT INFORMATION:

Law Office of Carolyn Buppert

1419 Forest Drive, Suite 205

Annapolis, MD 21403

Telephone (443) 482-3360

Web site: www.buppert.com